YOGA

PRACTICING POSTURES

An **EASY-TO-USE** Workbook

CONNIE WEISS

FIRST EDITION
LURIE LANE PUBLISHING
MORRO BAY, CALIFORNIA

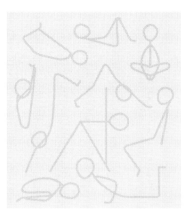

Copyright © 1991 by Connie Weiss

Printed in the United States of America.

LURIE LANE PUBLISHING
P.O. Box 893
Morro Bay, California 93442

ILLUSTRATIONS, TYPESETTING & PAGE PRODUCTION
Philah Graphics, Los Osos, California

COVERS AND SEGMENT DIVIDER DESIGN
Aldridge Design, Cambria, California

AUTHOR PHOTO
Darren Westlund, Cambria, California

ISBN 0-9629676-0-2

HAAGEN PRINTING • SANTA BARBARA • CALIFORNIA

TABLE OF CONTENTS

ACKNOWLEDGEMENTS

The author wishes to thank:

Katrina Rosa who in asking me to write a proposal on stress management set this long-germinating project in motion.

Barbara Garn of Philah Graphics who took on the project of making the book and drawings camera ready and found herself enmeshed in the world of the "little people" practicing postures. Untold hours later her artistry and her Macintosh computer have created living line drawings and a lovely milieu of font and space in which they exist.

Susan Aldridge for her cover and segment divider designs. Her directness and calm assertiveness made working with her a pleasure.

Peter Diffley for his patience, support and ability to edit, even in a language that was very foreign to him.

Karen Williams for her enthusiasm and persistence in wading through an early version of this book and for her advice concerning the arrangement of postures.

Karen Perault, whose editorial skills honed the non-postural portions of this book.

Melanie Callahan, Shoosh Crotzer, Dr. Robin Peterson, Katrina Rosa and Sandy Young for their encouragement and advice in describing postures and proof-reading the manuscript.

Ed Zolkoski for his helpful advice concerning the publication of this book.

And the lady with the gentle, resonating voice, Lolly Grafton, who was so responsive in representing Haagen Printing.

PREFACE

Over the twenty years that I have been leading yoga classes, my students have complained that they tried to practice at home, but couldn't remember the postures and their sequences ("what to do when"). And, while many yoga books offer insight into the philosophy of yoga and describe the forms of postures, sequencing has generally been relegated to lists of postures. The reader must page through an index and/or book to find postures, sometimes named in sanskrit. Believing that such a process is unnecessarily difficult, I have devised this easy-to-follow manual for people of all flexibility levels to facilitate individual practice sessions.

An array of safely ordered postures is presented so that you can vary your practice. Variety will help ensure that your attention will stay focused upon each moment of each posture; and it is ATTENTION that is of the utmost importance in achieving the mental and physical benefits of yoga and minimizing the risks of injury.

It is my hope that this book will be useful to you, alone or as an adjunct to classes, until you feel fully confident in devising your own practice sessions.

Namaste
(The spirit within me salutes the spirit within you.)

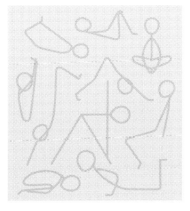

INTRODUCTION

I was introduced to yoga and inspired to practice by Eleanore Pagenstecher, a lady more than twice my age and twice my energy level.

My Teacher's Certificate was earned after study with "Mataji" Indra Devi, that world renowned Lady of Yoga whose vitality and longevity provide an incredible role model. I still remember the glee in her eye and the bemused look on her face as "oohs and aahs" filled the room at Rancho Cachuma in Tecate, Mexico in response to the sharp slap of her feet on the floor as she demonstrated how to fall from an imbalanced headstand safely. She was 75 at the time.

Several years later I worked (and I do not use the word lightly) in the Iyengar tradition with Kesheva (Jay) Kronish. I was challenged to achieve the precise alignment dictated for each posture and to develop the strength and endurance to remain in the poses.

Most recently I have been influenced by T.K.V. Desikachar and Professor A.G. Mohan. From them I have learned more about sequencing, using the breath to modify the postures and performing the postures dynamically.

Some of the postures in this book may remind you, as they do me, of their derivation. For example, the progression of seated legs-wide-apart postures and then bridging (page 63) was suggested to me by masseuse and Rolfer, Margaret Soulé-Eyles. The forming of an "O" hand exercise (page 77) came from Eve Cherry in an Arthritis Self-Help Class. The head turn movement leading with the energy body (page 80) is from a workshop with Richard Miller. Other postures are an amalgam, formed from numerous classes, workshops and teachers.

Finally, I want to recognize the people who have participated in class with me; being with you has given me much joy and satisfaction; watching and working with you has given me a greater understanding of the postures and the process.

With deep gratitude, I thank all of my teachers, including the many who have not been named. It has been and continues to be a fascinating path.

Connie Weiss
Morro Bay, California, 1991

READ BEFORE YOU PRACTICE

1   **If you have any health concerns, consult a yoga professional and/or your physician before you begin practicing the postures in this book.**

2   DEFINITIONS AND EXPLANATIONS

SEGMENT: a group of routines (Segment 1: Standing Postures, Segment II: Kneeling Postures; Segment III: Supine Postures; Segment IV: Prone Postures, Segment V: Seated Postures).

ROUTINE: a page of postures (asanas) in a segment (or less than a page, according to the instructions at the beginning of the segment).

In lieu of page numbers, each posture is identified in the lower right hand corner, thus: II.3.**5**; segment, routine, posture.

PRACTICE SESSION:
1. One routine from each of the five segments, plus Savasana, final relaxation, or
2. Practice Session Against the Wall, page 85, or
3. Sun Salutation, page 82, or Modified Sun Salutation, page 83.
4. For other options: see Introduction to Segment I, page 13, and Introduction to Segment II, page 27.

3   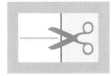 **THIS BOOK IS DESIGNED SO THAT YOU CAN CUT ON THE LINES BETWEEN POSTURES.** Once you have separated the postures you will be able to arrange postures from different pages in that segment to form different routines. In other words, all #1 postures in a segment can be interchanged with one another, all #2 postures in a segment can be interchanged with one another, etc., unless otherwise indicated. (If you choose not to cut your book, you can make the same choices with a bit more page flipping.)

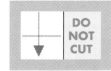 Do not cut between postures where an arrow indicates that one posture should follow another.

READ BEFORE YOU PRACTICE

4   To familiarize yourself with this book, read all of the segment introductions before you begin to practice.

5   Do not practice for 1½ hours after you have eaten. The time after a larger meal should be 3-4 hours. You may eat ½ hour after you have completed your practice.

6   To practice, begin with Segment I and follow the instructions for each segment.

7   To practice a posture, first study the picture and the words. Every posture has a beginning, a middle, and an end. Visualize the entire posture before you try to perform it.

8   **If a posture is described for the right side, always repeat on the left side.** The direction **round** means: do the right side and then the left side.

9   • OPTION: There are options given for some postures. Try those that are appropriate for your flexibility level.

10   ⓒ Indicates postures that can be modified and practiced while seated on a straight chair without arms. Place feet flat on floor, hip-width apart.

11   Ⓗ Indicates postures that can be held to create variety and increase intensity. Hold a pose as long as it is comfortable and of interest to you. Breathing should continue while the pose is held.

12   Frequently you can move directly from one pose to another. In other sequences you will want to extend your legs in between postures.

CONTINUED NEXT PAGE

READ BEFORE YOU PRACTICE

13 Remember that you can stop and rest as you need to during each practice, no matter where you are in an asana progression. The **major "back rest" positions** are **lying on your back with your knees folded to your chest** and the **Child Pose (II.1.1).** Assume one of these postures whenever necessary. You are your best teacher. **Listen to your body.**

14 Be aware of the sensations of pain. "Sweet Pain" may be experienced when stretching but your breath will be unimpeded. **"Sour Pain" must be avoided.** It is counter-productive, creating tightness, tension and fear in your body. If you do not heed the warning of pain your body could take many months to heal.

15 Never bounce as you stretch.

16 **Pay attention to your breath.** Breathe as slowly and as deeply as you can. Do not create tension within your body from overly extending the length of your inhalation or your exhalation.

17 Inhale and exhale through your nose, if possible.

18 If your breath becomes labored or erratic you are working too hard. Stop and rest until your breath normalizes.

19 **Exhale as you fold forward and as you twist.**
Inhale as you open and expand your body.

20 I have given the sanskrit names for many postures so that you can easily cross-reference to other sources for more detailed descriptions of them. In some cases the English translations, as well as the sanskrit names, vary from tradition to tradition.

SEGMENT I STANDING POSTURES

■ The practice of standing postures will warm your body and increase your strength and stability.

■ Practice the postures in this segment in order, 1-6. Remember, you may interchange any #1 posture in this segment with any other #1 posture in this segment, similarily for numbers 2, 3, 4, 5 and 6.

■ You may choose to do only the first 3 postures in any of these routines if you are limited in energy or time. If you do go beyond #3 posture, continue through #6.

■ Sun Salutations (pgs. 82-83) are an optional addition to this segment.

■ For variety, omit Segment I and begin with Segment II.

Raising Arms from Front

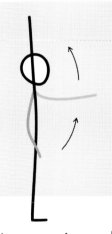

Arms alongside body, backs of hands face forward. Leading with backs of hands raise arms in front of you and up to the ceiling.

Raising Arms from Side

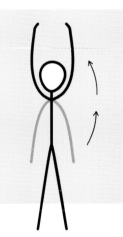

Arms alongside body, palms facing sides of thighs. Leading with backs of hands raise arms to the sides, right and left. At about shoulder level rotate arms so palms face upward. Continue to raise arms; palms face each other over head.

As you raise and lower arms keep fingers, wrists and elbows relaxed. When arms are over head, elbows can be bent but try to keep arms aligned with ears.

When we get hurt practicing postures it is either due to inattention or greed.

■ JOEL KRAMER
Workshop at Larchmont Center for Yoga,1981

TO BEGIN

1   Stand with your feet a few inches apart; allow them to turn open to the sides slightly so that you have a sense of stability.

2   Balance your weight between the heels and the balls of your feet.

3   Balance your weight between your right leg and your left leg.

4   Let your knees bend slightly.

5   Release your belly.

6   Gently lift your chest and let your shoulders roll back and down (keep your belly soft).

7   Lengthen your neck and let your head center on it.

8   Relax your eyes (open or closed).

9   Without changing it, take notice of your breath. Where is it moving in your body? What is the length of your inhalation? What is the length of your exhalation?

10 Once you have noted exactly how you are, you are ready to continue your practice. You have a template on which to register each posture and each breath. Stop your sequence now and then to do exactly the same thing... find out how you are... where you are breathing. (Remember that there is no right. There is no wrong. There simply is: watch without judging.)

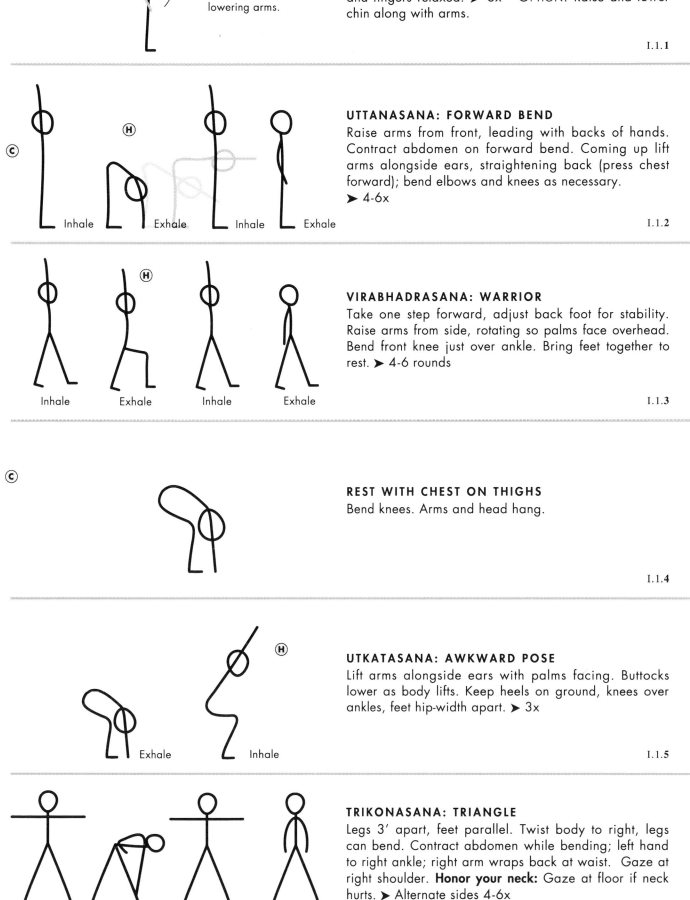

Ⓒ

TADASANA = SAMASTHITI: MOUNTAIN POSE
Stand erect, tuck chin to throat; raise and lower arms from front, leading up with backs of hands; keep wrists and fingers relaxed. ➤ 6x • OPTION: Raise and lower chin along with arms.

Inhale raising arms; exhale lowering arms.

I.1.**1**

Ⓒ

Inhale Exhale Inhale Exhale

UTTANASANA: FORWARD BEND
Raise arms from front, leading with backs of hands. Contract abdomen on forward bend. Coming up lift arms alongside ears, straightening back (press chest forward); bend elbows and knees as necessary.
➤ 4-6x

I.1.**2**

Inhale Exhale Inhale Exhale

VIRABHADRASANA: WARRIOR
Take one step forward, adjust back foot for stability. Raise arms from side, rotating so palms face overhead. Bend front knee just over ankle. Bring feet together to rest. ➤ 4-6 rounds

I.1.**3**

Ⓒ

REST WITH CHEST ON THIGHS
Bend knees. Arms and head hang.

I.1.**4**

Exhale Inhale

UTKATASANA: AWKWARD POSE
Lift arms alongside ears with palms facing. Buttocks lower as body lifts. Keep heels on ground, knees over ankles, feet hip-width apart. ➤ 3x

I.1.**5**

Inhale Exhale Inhale coming up. Exhale. Release.

TRIKONASANA: TRIANGLE
Legs 3' apart, feet parallel. Twist body to right, legs can bend. Contract abdomen while bending; left hand to right ankle; right arm wraps back at waist. Gaze at right shoulder. **Honor your neck:** Gaze at floor if neck hurts. ➤ Alternate sides 4-6x

I.1.**6**

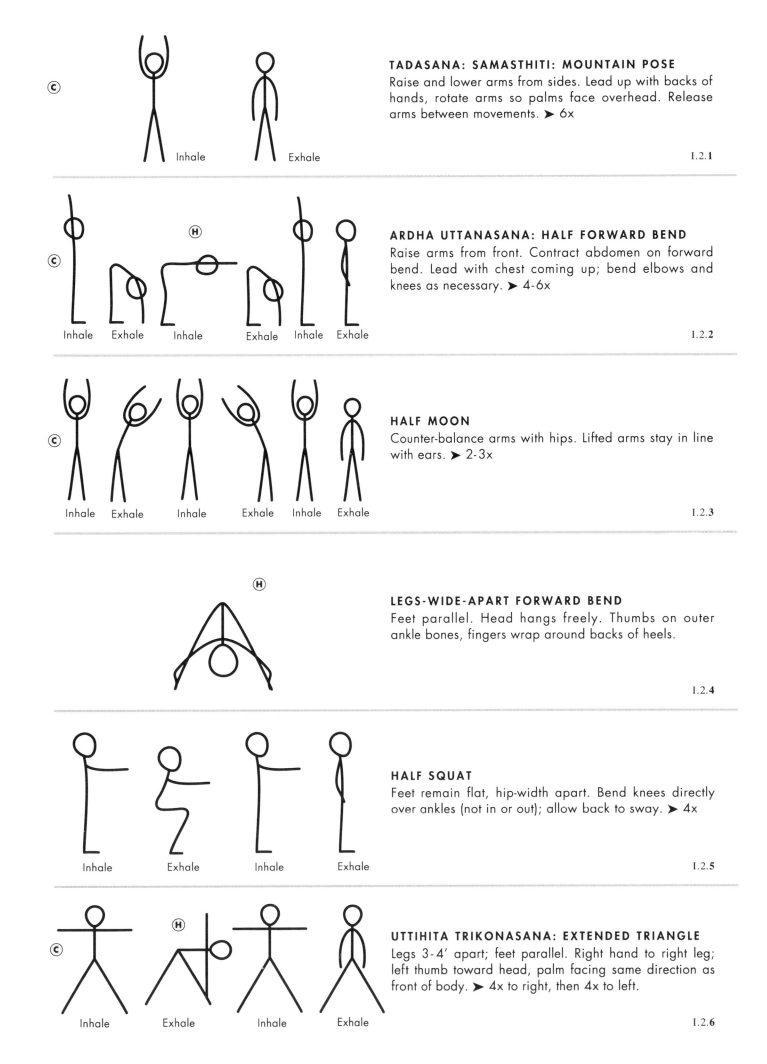

TADASANA: SAMASTHITI: MOUNTAIN POSE
Raise and lower arms from sides. Lead up with backs of hands, rotate arms so palms face overhead. Release arms between movements. ➤ 6x

Inhale   Exhale

I.2.1

ARDHA UTTANASANA: HALF FORWARD BEND
Raise arms from front. Contract abdomen on forward bend. Lead with chest coming up; bend elbows and knees as necessary. ➤ 4-6x

Inhale   Exhale   Inhale   Exhale   Inhale   Exhale

I.2.2

HALF MOON
Counter-balance arms with hips. Lifted arms stay in line with ears. ➤ 2-3x

Inhale   Exhale   Inhale   Exhale   Inhale   Exhale

I.2.3

LEGS-WIDE-APART FORWARD BEND
Feet parallel. Head hangs freely. Thumbs on outer ankle bones, fingers wrap around backs of heels.

I.2.4

HALF SQUAT
Feet remain flat, hip-width apart. Bend knees directly over ankles (not in or out); allow back to sway. ➤ 4x

Inhale   Exhale   Inhale   Exhale

I.2.5

UTTIHITA TRIKONASANA: EXTENDED TRIANGLE
Legs 3-4' apart; feet parallel. Right hand to right leg; left thumb toward head, palm facing same direction as front of body. ➤ 4x to right, then 4x to left.

Inhale   Exhale   Inhale   Exhale

I.2.6

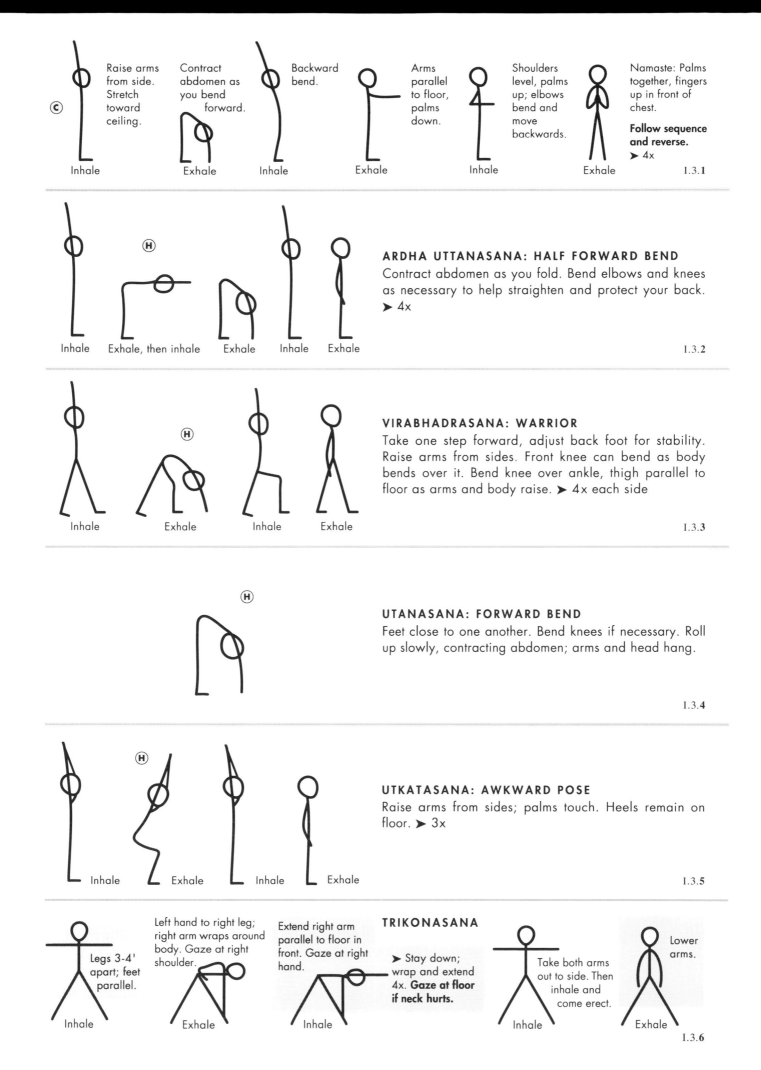

© Raise arms from side. Stretch toward ceiling.
Inhale

Contract abdomen as you bend forward.
Exhale

Backward bend.
Inhale

Arms parallel to floor, palms down.
Exhale

Shoulders level, palms up; elbows bend and move backwards.
Inhale

Namaste: Palms together, fingers up in front of chest.
Follow sequence and reverse.
➤ 4x
Exhale

I.3.1

Inhale   Exhale, then inhale   Exhale   Inhale   Exhale

ARDHA UTTANASANA: HALF FORWARD BEND
Contract abdomen as you fold. Bend elbows and knees as necessary to help straighten and protect your back.
➤ 4x

I.3.2

Inhale   Exhale   Inhale   Exhale

VIRABHADRASANA: WARRIOR
Take one step forward, adjust back foot for stability. Raise arms from sides. Front knee can bend as body bends over it. Bend knee over ankle, thigh parallel to floor as arms and body raise. ➤ 4x each side

I.3.3

UTANASANA: FORWARD BEND
Feet close to one another. Bend knees if necessary. Roll up slowly, contracting abdomen; arms and head hang.

I.3.4

Inhale   Exhale   Inhale   Exhale

UTKATASANA: AWKWARD POSE
Raise arms from sides; palms touch. Heels remain on floor. ➤ 3x

I.3.5

Legs 3-4' apart; feet parallel.
Inhale

Left hand to right leg; right arm wraps around body. Gaze at right shoulder.
Exhale

Extend right arm parallel to floor in front. Gaze at right hand.
Inhale

TRIKONASANA
➤ Stay down; wrap and extend 4x. **Gaze at floor if neck hurts.**

Take both arms out to side. Then inhale and come erect.
Inhale

Lower arms.
Exhale

I.3.6

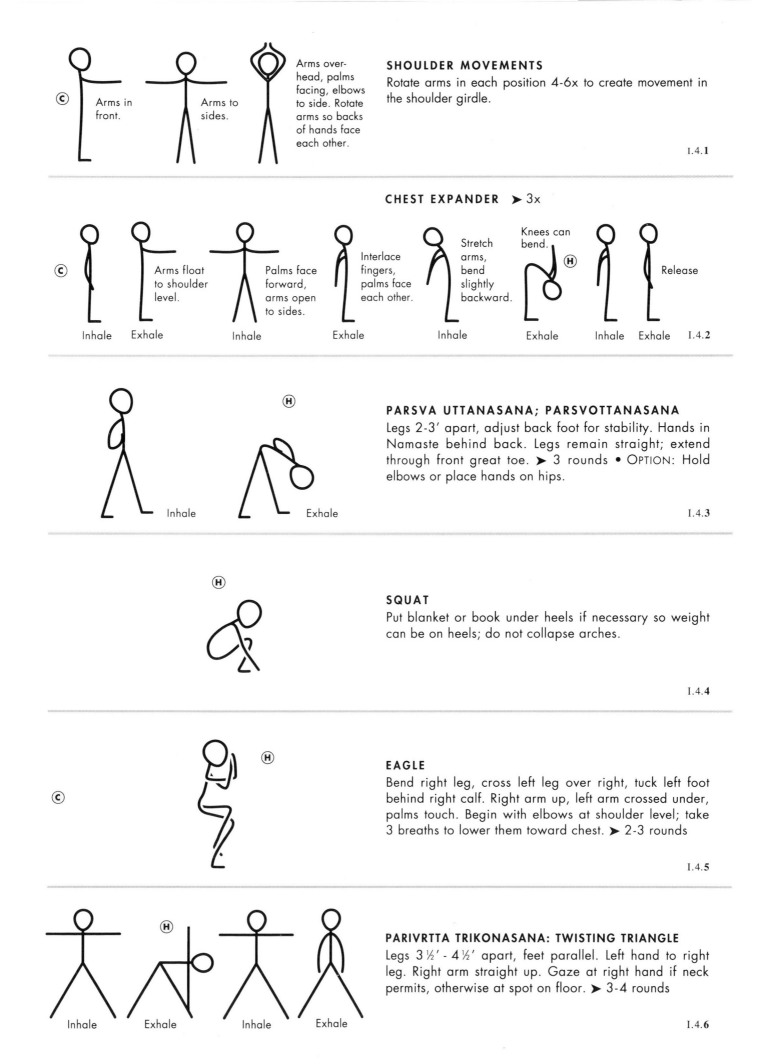

SHOULDER MOVEMENTS

Rotate arms in each position 4-6x to create movement in the shoulder girdle.

© Arms in front.

Arms to sides.

Arms overhead, palms facing, elbows to side. Rotate arms so backs of hands face each other.

I.4.1

CHEST EXPANDER ➤ 3x

© Inhale

Arms float to shoulder level. Exhale

Palms face forward, arms open to sides. Inhale

Interlace fingers, palms face each other. Exhale

Stretch arms, bend slightly backward. Inhale

Knees can bend. Ⓗ Exhale

Inhale

Release Exhale I.4.2

PARSVA UTTANASANA; PARSVOTTANASANA

Legs 2-3' apart, adjust back foot for stability. Hands in Namaste behind back. Legs remain straight; extend through front great toe. ➤ 3 rounds • OPTION: Hold elbows or place hands on hips.

Ⓗ

Inhale

Exhale

I.4.3

SQUAT

Put blanket or book under heels if necessary so weight can be on heels; do not collapse arches.

Ⓗ

I.4.4

EAGLE

Bend right leg, cross left leg over right, tuck left foot behind right calf. Right arm up, left arm crossed under, palms touch. Begin with elbows at shoulder level; take 3 breaths to lower them toward chest. ➤ 2-3 rounds

© Ⓗ

I.4.5

PARIVRTTA TRIKONASANA: TWISTING TRIANGLE

Legs 3½' - 4½' apart, feet parallel. Left hand to right leg. Right arm straight up. Gaze at right hand if neck permits, otherwise at spot on floor. ➤ 3-4 rounds

Inhale Exhale Ⓗ Inhale Exhale

I.4.6

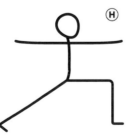

VRKSASANA: TREE

Place right foot on left thigh, open knee to side; arms overhead, palms touch or hands in Namaste (palms together, fingers up in front of chest). • OPTION: Lift right foot off floor and balance with knee pointed forward.

I.5.**1**

FORWARD BEND

Feet parallel, about 2' apart. Bend knees as you come upright (keep weight in your thighs to protect your back).

I.5.**2**

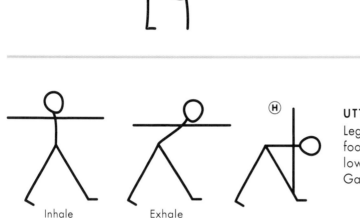

Inhale Exhale

UTTIHITA TRIKONASANA: EXTENDED TRIANGLE

Legs 3 ½' - 4 ½' apart. Open right foot to right, turn left foot slightly to right. Reach to right as hips move left; lower right hand to right leg while raising left hand. Gaze at left hand if neck permits. ➤ 3 rounds

I.5.**3**

FORWARD BEND

Feet parallel, hip-width apart. Hold elbows with opposite hands. Pull arms back alongside ears. Let head hang.

I.5.**4**

VIRABHADRASANA II

Legs 3 ½' - 4 ½' apart. Open right foot to right, turn left foot slightly to right. Extend arms to side parallel to floor. Bend right knee directly over ankle, thigh parallel to floor. Keep torso centered between legs; gaze over right hand. ➤ 2-3 rounds

I.5.**5**

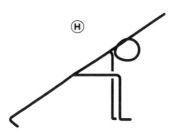

UTTHITA PARSVAKONASANA: EXTENDED LATERAL TRIANGLE

Legs 3 ½' - 4 ½' apart. Bend right knee over ankle, thigh parallel to floor. Place right hand on floor outside right foot. Extend left arm along left cheek. Gaze to ceiling under left upper arm. Extend through body from left foot to left hand. ➤ 2-3 rounds

I.5.**6**

SEGMENT II KNEELING POSTURES

■ The practice of postures in this segment will warm and stretch your spine and hips, help develop and maintain strength in your arms and suppleness in your shoulders. Many of these postures encourage full deep breathing.

■ Practice the postures in this segment in order 1-6, interchanging like-numbered postures from different routines as you wish. Note that II.6.1. and II.6.2. are paired.

■ You may exclude posture #4 from all routines in this segment, but do conclude your routine with posture #5, the Child Pose.

■ **If you have difficulty kneeling** any of the following may help:

1 Fold a blanket and place it behind your knees to create enough space between your upper and lower legs so that your knees don't hurt when you sit back on your heels.

2 Place a blanket or mat under your knees for the all fours position (p.83) or kneeling.

3 Place a rolled towel under your insteps if they are stiff.

4 If you say "no way," adapt postures marked " Ⓒ " for chair use in place of kneeling postures. The Board and Downward Facing Dog should be fine for most people.

■ For variety, or when you feel particularly tired, omit this segment (even if you have also omitted Segment I) and go on to Segment III (p. 41).

We must always choose the hat to fit the head; not choose the hat and make the head fit it. The same is true for yoga postures.

■ PROFESSOR A.G. MOHAN
Workshop at Meadowlark, 1989

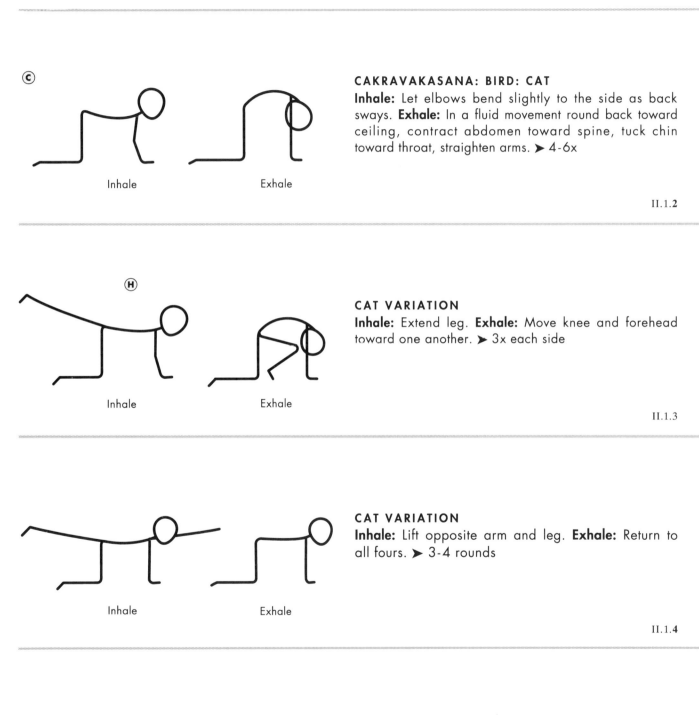

CHILD POSE

Arms are like empty coatsleeves alongside body, backs of hands on floor. If you feel too much pressure in your head, make fists of your hands, placing one on top of the other vertically and placing your forehead on top of them.

II.1.**1**

CAKRAVAKASANA: BIRD: CAT

Inhale: Let elbows bend slightly to the side as back sways. **Exhale:** In a fluid movement round back toward ceiling, contract abdomen toward spine, tuck chin toward throat, straighten arms. ➤ 4-6x

Inhale

Exhale

II.1.**2**

CAT VARIATION

Inhale: Extend leg. **Exhale:** Move knee and forehead toward one another. ➤ 3x each side

Inhale

Exhale

II.1.3

CAT VARIATION

Inhale: Lift opposite arm and leg. **Exhale:** Return to all fours. ➤ 3-4 rounds

Inhale

Exhale

II.1.**4**

CHILD POSE

Arms alongside body, backs of hands on floor. Roll from thumb to little finger across backs of hands; will release wrists.

II.1.5

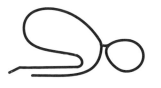

WIDE-KNEED CHILD POSE
Knees well apart, belly between thighs; shoulders to floor; cheek or forehead to floor.

II.2.**1**

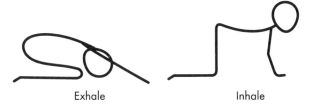

Exhale   Inhale

CAKRAVAKASANA: CAT
Knees and feet hip-width apart. Fold back, then glide to cat; bend elbows slightly. ➤ 4-6x

II.2.**2**

ⓒ

Inhale   Exhale

VAJRASANA
Raise arms from front toward ceiling and come to upright kneeling position. Contract abdomen and fold chest toward thighs. Wrap arms around back and place forehead on floor. Exhale as slowly as possible. ➤ 4-6x

II.2.**3**

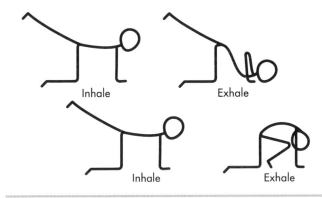

Inhale   Exhale

Inhale   Exhale

CAT VARIATION
Inhale: Lift leg. **Exhale:** Lower chest to floor as elbows bend off floor alongside body. **Inhale:** Come up as you went down; if that is not possible do not go down all the way. **Exhale:** Bring knee toward forehead. ➤ 3-4 rounds

II.2.**4**

ⓒ

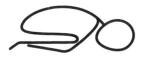

CHILD POSE
Shrug shoulders, then roll them down and away from your ears.

II.2.**5**

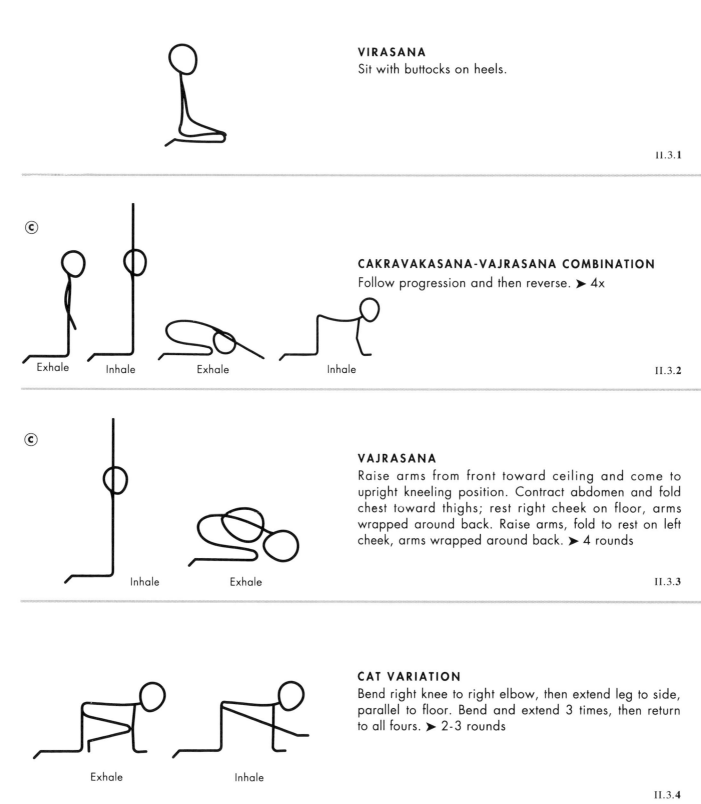

VIRASANA
Sit with buttocks on heels.

II.3.**1**

Ⓒ

CAKRAVAKASANA-VAJRASANA COMBINATION
Follow progression and then reverse. ➤ 4x

Exhale   Inhale   Exhale   Inhale

II.3.**2**

Ⓒ

VAJRASANA
Raise arms from front toward ceiling and come to upright kneeling position. Contract abdomen and fold chest toward thighs; rest right cheek on floor, arms wrapped around back. Raise arms, fold to rest on left cheek, arms wrapped around back. ➤ 4 rounds

Inhale   Exhale

II.3.**3**

CAT VARIATION
Bend right knee to right elbow, then extend leg to side, parallel to floor. Bend and extend 3 times, then return to all fours. ➤ 2-3 rounds

Exhale   Inhale

II.3.**4**

CHILD POSE
Keep buttocks on heels. Place palms together overhead, outer borders of hands on floor. Stretch arms and let elbows lift off floor.

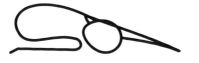

II.3.**5**

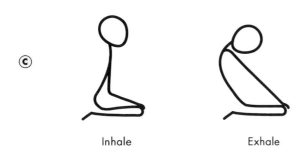

ⓒ

CAT
Sit on heels, hands on knees. Arch and then round back while sitting on heels. ➤ 4x

Inhale   Exhale

II.4.**1**

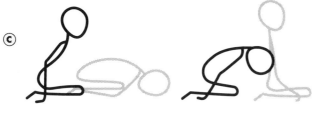

ⓒ

MOVING CHILD
Sit on heels. Arch back and fold to floor, leading with chest. Tuck chin to throat, contract abdomen and roll up with rounded back. Backs of hands on floor throughout. ➤ 4-6x

Exhale   Inhale

II.4.**2**

Ⓗ

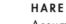

HARE
Assume Child Pose. Arms straight alongside body, thumbs on outer ankle bones, fingers wrap heels. Top of head on floor. Lift buttocks, roll head as if neck would move to floor. Feel stretch across upper back. ➤ 2-3x

II.4.**3**

Ⓗ

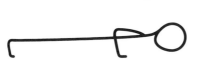

FOUR POINTS TOUCHING
Bend elbows, place hands on floor under shoulders, toes tucked. Press hands to floor, elbows hug body; lift legs, torso and head. Look down. Keep body straight. ➤ 2-3x

II.4.**4**

ⓒ

CHILD POSE
Feel the breath moving through your back as you inhale and exhale.

II.4.**5**

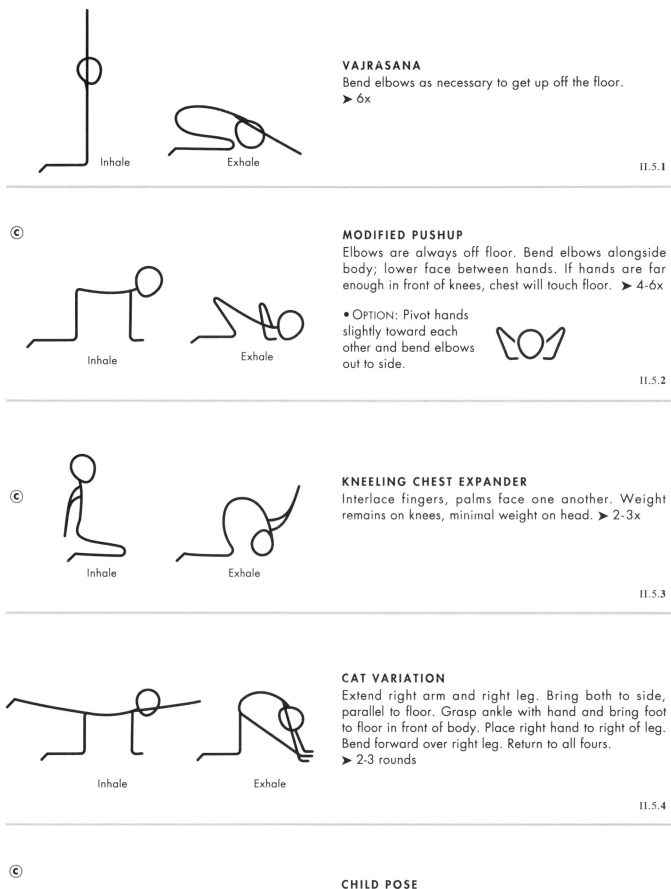

VAJRASANA

Bend elbows as necessary to get up off the floor.
➤ 6x

Inhale   Exhale

II.5.**1**

ⓒ

MODIFIED PUSHUP

Elbows are always off floor. Bend elbows alongside body; lower face between hands. If hands are far enough in front of knees, chest will touch floor. ➤ 4-6x

• OPTION: Pivot hands slightly toward each other and bend elbows out to side.

Inhale   Exhale

II.5.**2**

ⓒ

KNEELING CHEST EXPANDER

Interlace fingers, palms face one another. Weight remains on knees, minimal weight on head. ➤ 2-3x

Inhale   Exhale

II.5.**3**

CAT VARIATION

Extend right arm and right leg. Bring both to side, parallel to floor. Grasp ankle with hand and bring foot to floor in front of body. Place right hand to right of leg. Bend forward over right leg. Return to all fours.
➤ 2-3 rounds

Inhale   Exhale

II.5.**4**

ⓒ

CHILD POSE

Arms alongside body, backs of hands on floor. Pretend that strings attach your fingers to the heels of your hands. Close your fingers to form a gentle fist, taking 3 full breaths. Only move on the exhalation. ➤ 3x

II.5.**5**

VIRASANA

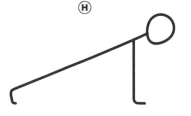

Buttocks on floor between heels. Toes point straight back. **Honor your knees.** Support yourself with your hands as necessary.

SUPTA VIRASANA

If possible, lean back, bend elbows and place forearms on floor. Then lower shoulders and head to floor. Hands grasp opposite elbows overhead. Bend elbows alongside body and lean into them to get up. **Honor your knees.**

If you do either of these poses, also do

II.6.**1**

BOARD POSITION

Fingers point straight ahead. Hands flat on floor shoulder-width apart. Toes tucked, straight legs. Posture will release knees after Virasana.

II.6.**2**

ADHOMUKHA SVANASANA: DOWNWARD FACING DOG

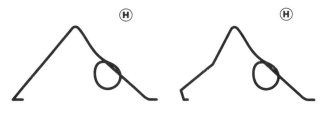

Fingers point straight ahead. Hands flat on floor shoulder-width apart. Press area between thumb and forefinger to floor. Bend elbows slightly if they hyperextend. Move chest toward thighs; roll sitz bones toward ceiling. Head hangs. ➤ Do several times or hold up to five breaths. • OPTION: Bend knees to get more extension through back.

II.6.**3**

BAKASANA: CRANE

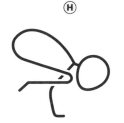

Bend elbows, rest knees on upper arms, balance on hands; feet off floor. ➤ 2-3x

II.6.**4**

CHILD POSE

Backs of hands on floor. Widen fingers, then make fists; will release wrists. Repeat several times.

II.6.**5**

SEGMENT III SUPINE POSTURES

■ The practice of the postures in this segment will help you collect yourself from external distractions and return to your "center."

■ The postures of routine 1 in this segment are invaluable for helping release stressed lower backs. Omit posture #5 if you are experiencing any lower back pain. In fact, avoid all twisting movements if your lower back is injured.

■ Practice the postures in this segment in order 1-6. As in other segments, you can vary your practice by interchanging like-numbered postures from different routines.

■ To begin, assume the savasana position (p. 75) for a few moments. Watch as your breath softens, your body quiets and your mind, your body and your breath all re-form a harmonious whole.

When we study yoga we begin where we are, as we are, and what happens, happens.

■ PROFESSOR A.G. MOHAN
Workshop at Meadowlark, 1990

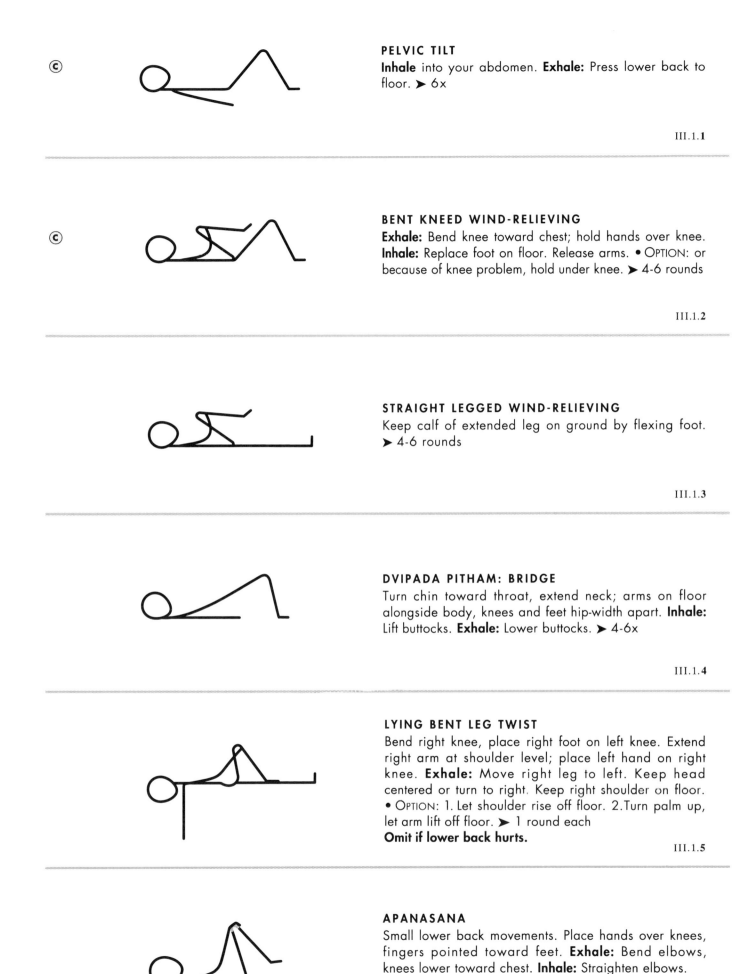

PELVIC TILT

Ⓒ

Inhale into your abdomen. **Exhale:** Press lower back to floor. ➤ 6x

III.1.**1**

BENT KNEED WIND-RELIEVING

Ⓒ

Exhale: Bend knee toward chest; hold hands over knee. **Inhale:** Replace foot on floor. Release arms. • OPTION: or because of knee problem, hold under knee. ➤ 4-6 rounds

III.1.**2**

STRAIGHT LEGGED WIND-RELIEVING

Keep calf of extended leg on ground by flexing foot. ➤ 4-6 rounds

III.1.**3**

DVIPADA PITHAM: BRIDGE

Turn chin toward throat, extend neck; arms on floor alongside body, knees and feet hip-width apart. **Inhale:** Lift buttocks. **Exhale:** Lower buttocks. ➤ 4-6x

III.1.**4**

LYING BENT LEG TWIST

Bend right knee, place right foot on left knee. Extend right arm at shoulder level; place left hand on right knee. **Exhale:** Move right leg to left. Keep head centered or turn to right. Keep right shoulder on floor. • OPTION: 1. Let shoulder rise off floor. 2. Turn palm up, let arm lift off floor. ➤ 1 round each
Omit if lower back hurts.

III.1.**5**

APANASANA

Small lower back movements. Place hands over knees, fingers pointed toward feet. **Exhale:** Bend elbows, knees lower toward chest. **Inhale:** Straighten elbows.

III.1.**6**

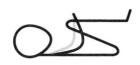

APANASANA

Interlace fingers and place hands over knees (or hold knees with hands). Roll from elbow to elbow across back.

III.2.**1**

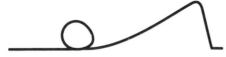

PUMP

Point toes. **Inhale:** Lift right leg to ceiling. **Exhale:** Flex foot, lead with heel to floor. Breathe the whole time the leg is moving. ➤ 4-6 rounds.

III.2.**2**

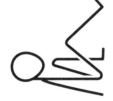

RAISED LEG POSE

Fold knees to chest. **Inhale:** Extend right leg toward ceiling. **Exhale:** Rebend. Do left leg. Then do both legs. Arms remain alongside body. • OPTION: Raise arms (singly or together) to floor overhead and down as legs move. ➤ 4-6 rounds

III.2.**3**

DVIPADA PITHAM: BRIDGE

Lift arms overhead as buttocks lift and lower as buttocks return to floor. **Inhale** up; **exhale** down. ➤ 4x

III.2.**4**

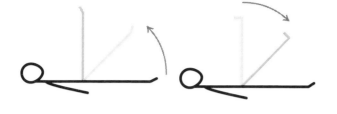

There are numerous counter-indications for practicing shoulder stands. Discuss your condition with a yoga professional and/or your physician.

HEADSTAND

➤ Practice before the shoulder stand and **only** if it is very easy for you or you've had formal instruction.

VIPARITAKARANI: MODIFIED SHOULDER STAND

Hold up to 24 breaths. Knees may bend slightly and legs may be slightly apart. **Honor your neck.**

III.2.**5**

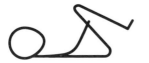

APANASANA

Place hands under knees. **Exhale:** Move knees toward chest. **Inhale:** Move knees slightly away from chest.

III.2.**6**

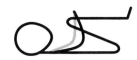

APANASANA

Interlace fingers and place hands over knees. Legs move 10° to right while head turns 10° to left; then reverse.

III.3.**1**

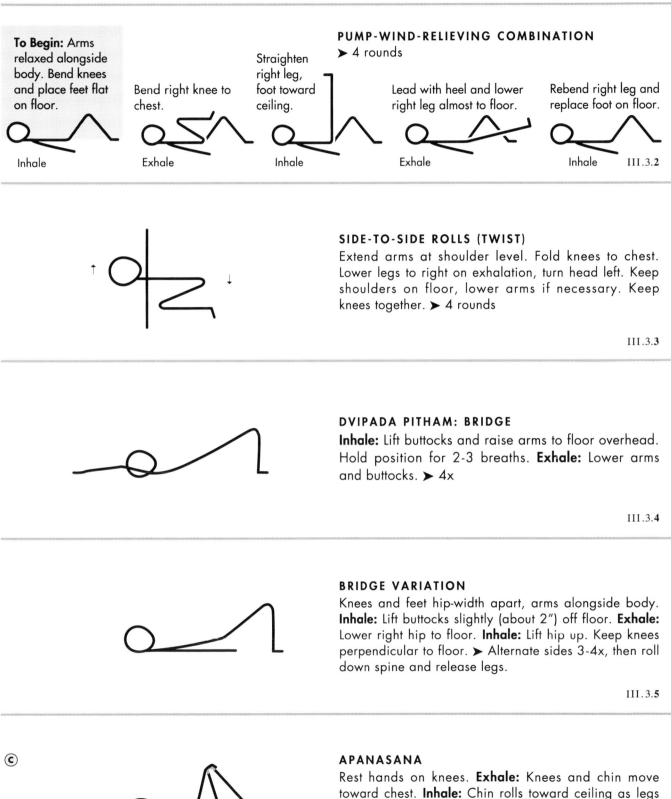

To Begin: Arms relaxed alongside body. Bend knees and place feet flat on floor.

PUMP-WIND-RELIEVING COMBINATION
➤ 4 rounds

Bend right knee to chest.

Straighten right leg, foot toward ceiling.

Lead with heel and lower right leg almost to floor.

Rebend right leg and replace foot on floor.

Inhale · Exhale · Inhale · Exhale · Inhale · III.3.**2**

SIDE-TO-SIDE ROLLS (TWIST)

Extend arms at shoulder level. Fold knees to chest. Lower legs to right on exhalation, turn head left. Keep shoulders on floor, lower arms if necessary. Keep knees together. ➤ 4 rounds

III.3.**3**

DVIPADA PITHAM: BRIDGE

Inhale: Lift buttocks and raise arms to floor overhead. Hold position for 2-3 breaths. **Exhale:** Lower arms and buttocks. ➤ 4x

III.3.**4**

BRIDGE VARIATION

Knees and feet hip-width apart, arms alongside body. **Inhale:** Lift buttocks slightly (about 2") off floor. **Exhale:** Lower right hip to floor. **Inhale:** Lift hip up. Keep knees perpendicular to floor. ➤ Alternate sides 3-4x, then roll down spine and release legs.

III.3.**5**

Ⓒ

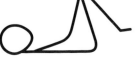

APANASANA

Rest hands on knees. **Exhale:** Knees and chin move toward chest. **Inhale:** Chin rolls toward ceiling as legs move away from chest. Feel breath expand and contract body.

III.3.**6**

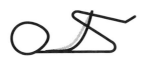

APANASANA

Massage back on floor. Hold knees with hands. Circle knees clockwise; pause; circle counterclockwise.

III.4.**1**

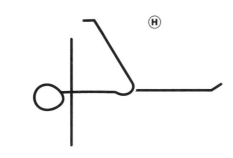

LYING TWIST

Bend arms and place fingers on shoulders. Legs 2' apart. Keep heels on floor as pivot points; roll over and put right elbow on floor near left elbow (head lifts). Return head and back to floor and roll across back to right, put left elbow to floor near right elbow. ➤ 3 rounds

III.4.**2**

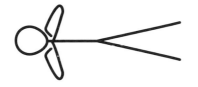

CROSSOVER TWIST

Point toes. **Inhale:** Right leg to ceiling. **Exhale:** Lower foot toward left hand, head turns to right. **Inhale:** Flex foot and roll straight leg to ceiling (modify by bending right knee at side and rolling to center) and head to center. **Exhale:** Lower right leg to floor alongside left leg. ➤ 3 rounds

III.4.**3**

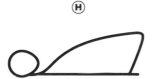

DVIPADA PITHAM: BRIDGE

Hold ankles with hands; knees and feet hip-width apart. ➤ 2-3x

III.4.**4**

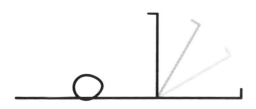

URDHVA PRASARITA PADASANA

Arms over head on floor. Lift both legs to 30°, 60° and 90° (holding at each level) and then lower slowly. **Keep lower back on floor throughout.** If back comes up, lift legs to next higher position immediately or, in lowering, immediately bend knees and put feet on the floor. **Keep breathing.**

III.4.**5**

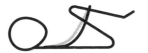

APANASANA

Fold knees to chest, interlace fingers and hold over knees. Roll from to side to side letting head move with rest of body.

III.4.**6**

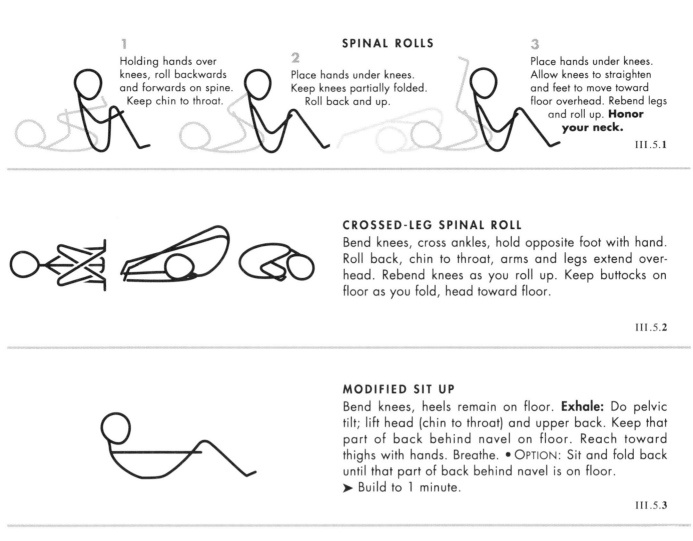

SPINAL ROLLS

1 Holding hands over knees, roll backwards and forwards on spine. Keep chin to throat.

2 Place hands under knees. Keep knees partially folded. Roll back and up.

3 Place hands under knees. Allow knees to straighten and feet to move toward floor overhead. Rebend legs and roll up. **Honor your neck.**

III.5.**1**

CROSSED-LEG SPINAL ROLL

Bend knees, cross ankles, hold opposite foot with hand. Roll back, chin to throat, arms and legs extend over-head. Rebend knees as you roll up. Keep buttocks on floor as you fold, head toward floor.

III.5.**2**

MODIFIED SIT UP

Bend knees, heels remain on floor. **Exhale:** Do pelvic tilt; lift head (chin to throat) and upper back. Keep that part of back behind navel on floor. Reach toward thighs with hands. Breathe. • OPTION: Sit and fold back until that part of back behind navel is on floor.

➤ Build to 1 minute.

III.5.**3**

BRIDGE VARIATION

➤ 2-3 rounds

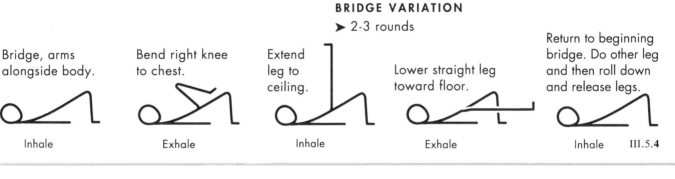

Bridge, arms alongside body.

Inhale

Bend right knee to chest.

Exhale

Extend leg to ceiling.

Inhale

Lower straight leg toward floor.

Exhale

Return to beginning bridge. Do other leg and then roll down and release legs.

Inhale III.5.**4**

SIDE LEG LIFTS

1 Lie on side. Bend bottom arm and support head with that hand, other arm straight in front of body. **Inhale:** Lift top leg, lead with outer ankle bone. Turn great toe downward (feel buttock). **Exhale:** Lower leg. ➤ 2-3x

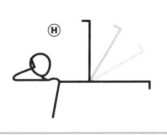

2 Rotate leg so toes face ceiling. **Inhale:** Lift leg (stretch inside of leg). **Exhale:** Lower leg, lead with heel. ➤ 2-3x

III.5.**5**

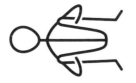

FLAT FROG

Fold knees toward armpits. Rest arms over lower legs, flattening back to floor.

III.5.**6**

SEGMENT IV PRONE POSTURES

■ Because we primarily bend forward in our daily activities, it is essential to practice backward-bending postures to maintain and improve the strength and flexibility of our backs.

■ Postures #1 and #6 are the same for all routines in this segment.

■ All #2 postures in this segment can be interchanged.

■ All #3 postures in this segment can be interchanged.

■ All #4 and #5 postures can be interchanged except for the Camel (IV.4.4.) and the Upward Bow (IV.4.5.) which are paired.

■ Watch your breath as you practice these postures. The pressure on your diaphragm coupled with the movements make breathing more difficult. Completely relax as necessary.

When you practice, the pose should be inside you, not you in the pose.

■ RICHARD MILLER
Workshop at Préma Vikára Yoga Center, 1990

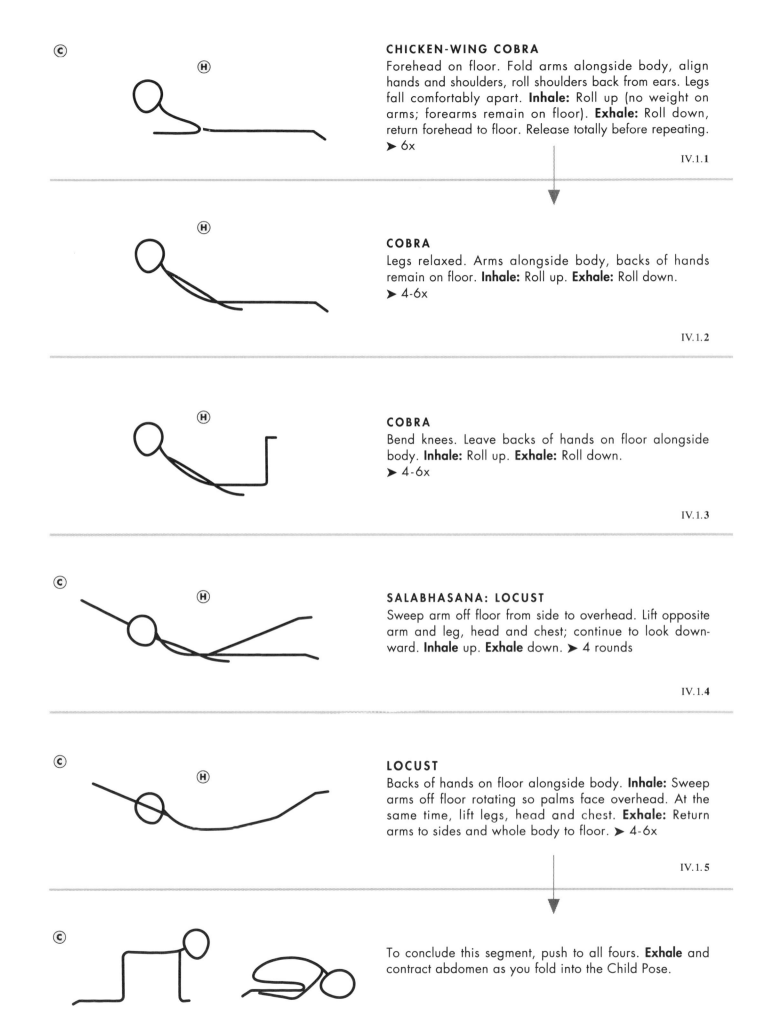

CHICKEN-WING COBRA
Forehead on floor. Fold arms alongside body, align hands and shoulders, roll shoulders back from ears. Legs fall comfortably apart. **Inhale:** Roll up (no weight on arms; forearms remain on floor). **Exhale:** Roll down, return forehead to floor. Release totally before repeating. ➤ 6x

IV.1.**1**

COBRA
Legs relaxed. Arms alongside body, backs of hands remain on floor. **Inhale:** Roll up. **Exhale:** Roll down. ➤ 4-6x

IV.1.**2**

COBRA
Bend knees. Leave backs of hands on floor alongside body. **Inhale:** Roll up. **Exhale:** Roll down. ➤ 4-6x

IV.1.**3**

SALABHASANA: LOCUST
Sweep arm off floor from side to overhead. Lift opposite arm and leg, head and chest; continue to look downward. **Inhale** up. **Exhale** down. ➤ 4 rounds

IV.1.**4**

LOCUST
Backs of hands on floor alongside body. **Inhale:** Sweep arms off floor rotating so palms face overhead. At the same time, lift legs, head and chest. **Exhale:** Return arms to sides and whole body to floor. ➤ 4-6x

IV.1.**5**

To conclude this segment, push to all fours. **Exhale** and contract abdomen as you fold into the Child Pose.

IV.1.**6**

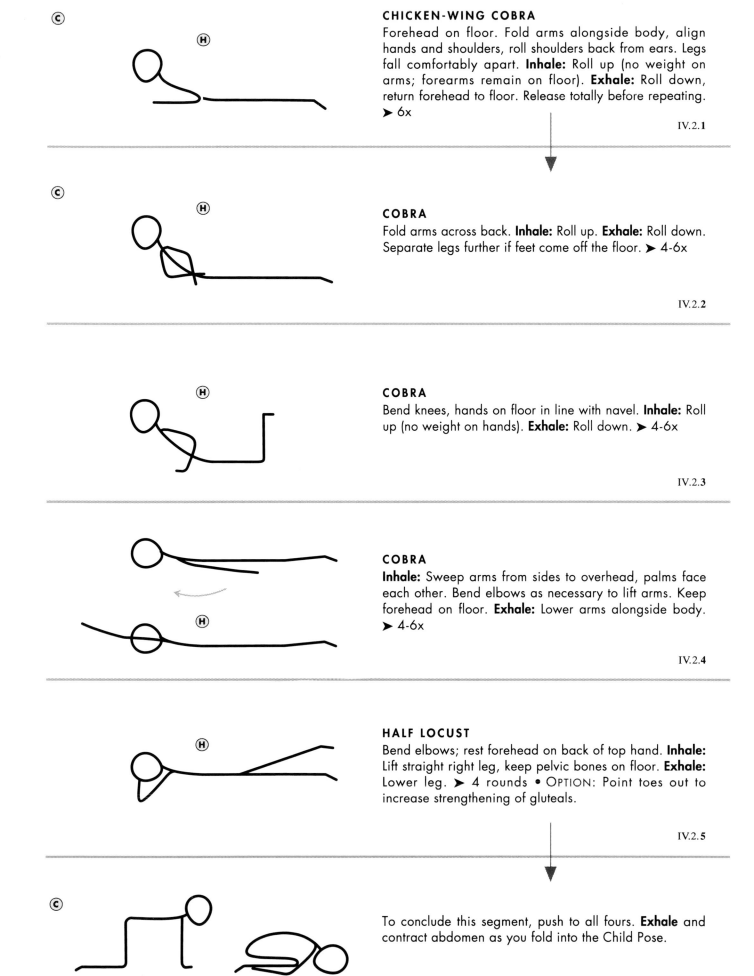

CHICKEN-WING COBRA

Forehead on floor. Fold arms alongside body, align hands and shoulders, roll shoulders back from ears. Legs fall comfortably apart. **Inhale:** Roll up (no weight on arms; forearms remain on floor). **Exhale:** Roll down, return forehead to floor. Release totally before repeating. ➤ 6x

IV.2.**1**

COBRA

Fold arms across back. **Inhale:** Roll up. **Exhale:** Roll down. Separate legs further if feet come off the floor. ➤ 4-6x

IV.2.**2**

COBRA

Bend knees, hands on floor in line with navel. **Inhale:** Roll up (no weight on hands). **Exhale:** Roll down. ➤ 4-6x

IV.2.**3**

COBRA

Inhale: Sweep arms from sides to overhead, palms face each other. Bend elbows as necessary to lift arms. Keep forehead on floor. **Exhale:** Lower arms alongside body. ➤ 4-6x

IV.2.**4**

HALF LOCUST

Bend elbows; rest forehead on back of top hand. **Inhale:** Lift straight right leg, keep pelvic bones on floor. **Exhale:** Lower leg. ➤ 4 rounds • OPTION: Point toes out to increase strengthening of gluteals.

IV.2.**5**

To conclude this segment, push to all fours. **Exhale** and contract abdomen as you fold into the Child Pose.

IV.2.**6**

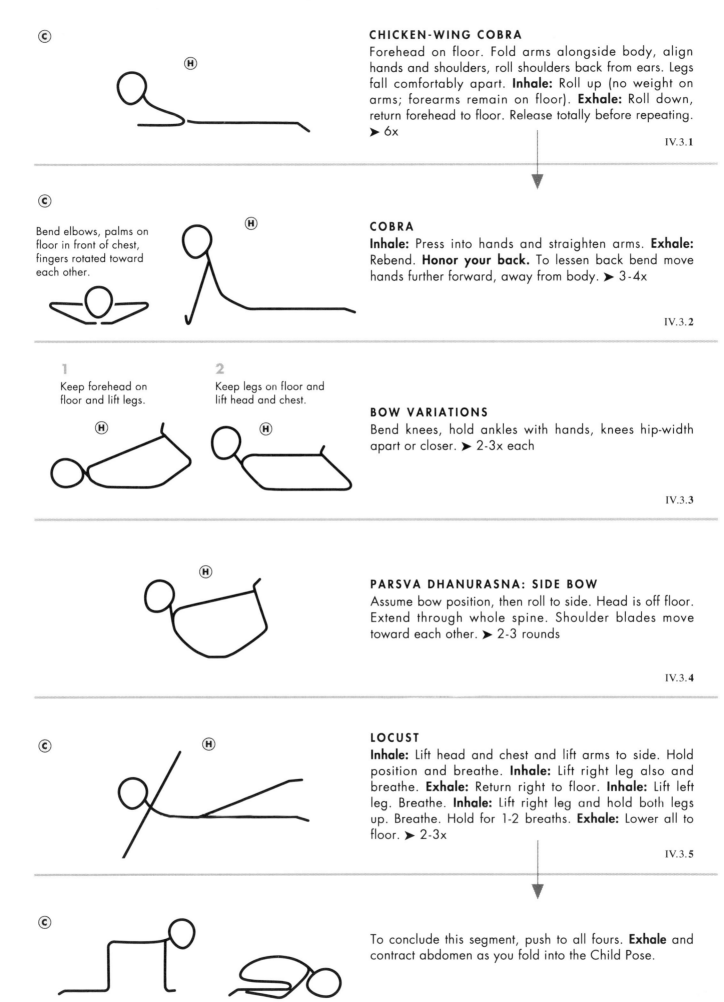

CHICKEN-WING COBRA

Forehead on floor. Fold arms alongside body, align hands and shoulders, roll shoulders back from ears. Legs fall comfortably apart. **Inhale:** Roll up (no weight on arms; forearms remain on floor). **Exhale:** Roll down, return forehead to floor. Release totally before repeating. ➤ 6x

IV.3.**1**

COBRA

Bend elbows, palms on floor in front of chest, fingers rotated toward each other.

Inhale: Press into hands and straighten arms. **Exhale:** Rebend. **Honor your back.** To lessen back bend move hands further forward, away from body. ➤ 3-4x

IV.3.**2**

1 Keep forehead on floor and lift legs.

2 Keep legs on floor and lift head and chest.

BOW VARIATIONS

Bend knees, hold ankles with hands, knees hip-width apart or closer. ➤ 2-3x each

IV.3.**3**

PARSVA DHANURASNA: SIDE BOW

Assume bow position, then roll to side. Head is off floor. Extend through whole spine. Shoulder blades move toward each other. ➤ 2-3 rounds

IV.3.**4**

LOCUST

Inhale: Lift head and chest and lift arms to side. Hold position and breathe. **Inhale:** Lift right leg also and breathe. **Exhale:** Return right to floor. **Inhale:** Lift left leg. Breathe. **Inhale:** Lift right leg and hold both legs up. Breathe. Hold for 1-2 breaths. **Exhale:** Lower all to floor. ➤ 2-3x

IV.3.**5**

To conclude this segment, push to all fours. **Exhale** and contract abdomen as you fold into the Child Pose.

IV.3.**6**

CHICKEN-WING COBRA

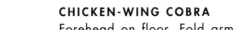

Forehead on floor. Fold arms alongside body, align hands and shoulders, roll shoulders back from ears. Legs fall comfortably apart. **Inhale:** Roll up (no weight on arms; forearms remain on floor). **Exhale:** Roll down, return forehead to floor. Release totally before repeating. ➤ 6x

IV.4.**1**

BHUJANGASANA: COBRA

Palms on floor, fingertips under shoulders, elbows off floor alongside body. **Inhale:** Curl up; roll shoulders away from ears, even when weight goes into hands. Always keep slight bend in elbows and pubic bone on floor. **Exhale:** Roll down. ➤ 2-3x

IV.4.**2**

DHANURASANA: BOW

Bend knees and grasp ankles with hands, knees hip-width apart. **Inhale** up. **Exhale** down. ➤ 2-3x
• OPTION: 1. Flex feet and close knees. 2. Do one leg at a time. (Bend right leg and grasp right ankle with right hand. Extend left arm on floor overhead. Leave left arm on floor as you lift right leg, head and chest.)
➤ 2-3 rounds

IV.4.**3**

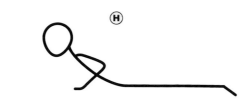

Tuck toes. Lift chest and extend spine, face forward

Roll shoulders back further and extend through whole spine as face turns toward ceiling (Do not just fold at juncture of two cervical vertebrae).

Toes flat, hands on soles of feet.

USTRASANA: CAMEL

Place thumbs on muscles on either side of spine just above hips to begin and raise from position. **Use Child Pose to release back.** ➤ 2-3x

If you do this pose, also do ⌐ (if possible).

IV.4.**4**

URDHVA DHANURASANA: UPWARD BOW

Bend elbows, place palms on floor, fingers under shoulders. Feet no further than hip-width apart. **Inhale:** Press hands, straighten arms, lift hips. Tuck chin to throat as head lowers to floor. ➤ 2-3x • OPTION: Come onto toes to further open upper back.

IV.4.**5**

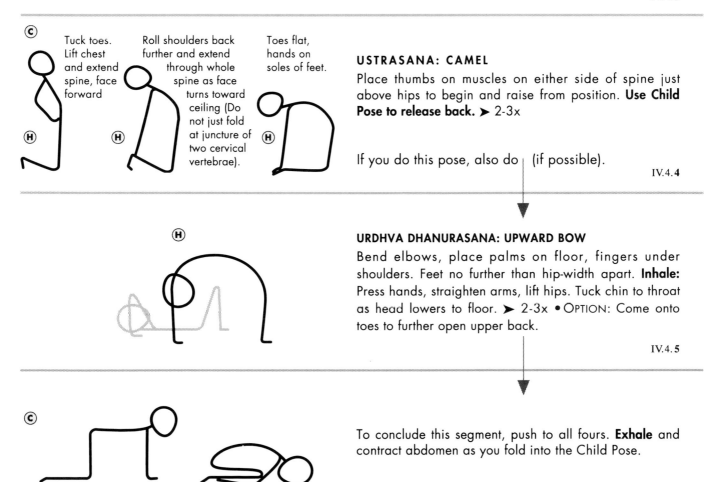

To conclude this segment, push to all fours. **Exhale** and contract abdomen as you fold into the Child Pose.

IV.4.**6**

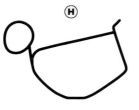

SEGMENT V SEATED POSTURES

■ The practice of the postures in this segment will stretch your arms, shoulders, torso, spine, legs and hips. Because many of the seated postures involve folding forward, in a sense closing up, they encourage introversion and will have a calming effect on your body and your mind.

■ Never bounce as you stretch.

■ Practice the postures in this segment in order 1-6. You may interchange like-numbered postures from routine to routine.

■ You may do more than one of the #2 legs-wide-apart postures when practicing any of these routines.

■ **Concerning legs-wide-apart postures:**

1 The purpose of these postures is the lateral stretch and the leg stretch. Do not be concerned if you cannot reach your toes.

2 To begin, sit on the floor and open your legs wide apart. Then use your hands to move the gluteals (muscles of the buttocks) backwards so the pelvis tips and the bottoms of the pelvic bones (SITZ BONES) are on the floor.

3 Following legs-wide-apart postures, tip back slightly on your buttocks, allowing your knees to give, and place your hands under your knees. Draw your knees into your chest and balance on your buttocks.

4 Then do Bridge, III.1.4., or Table, V.3.4., to reestablish the normal alignment of the lower back and pelvis.

The ultimate gift of yoga practice is that we become aware that we are not the body. We are the watchers...the part that is aware.

■ RICHARD MILLER
Workshop at Préma Vikára Yoga Center, 1990

PARVATASANA

Inhale: Lift arms from sides, palms up. Interlace fingers, turn palms to ceiling, stretch. Lift shoulders toward ears. Breathe. Lower shoulders. Breathe. Release fingers and lower arms slowly, inhaling and exhaling; feel air on palms of hands.

V.1.**1**

GOMUKHASANA: COWHEAD

Bend right knee and sit on right instep with one cheek of buttocks on each side of heel. Cross left leg over right knee. Place back of left hand on spine, fingers toward head. Lift right arm toward ceiling, bend elbow and grasp left hand with right. After releasing, extend arms to side slightly off floor palms facing forward, stretch.
• OPTION: Hold a towel between your hands if you cannot grasp hands.

V.1.**2**

DYNAMIC PASCHIMOTTANASANA

Inhale: Raise arms, lift chest, arch back. **Exhale:** Fold forward; let back round, head hang, knees bend.
➤ 4-6x

V.1.**3**

TWISTS ➤ Choose one:

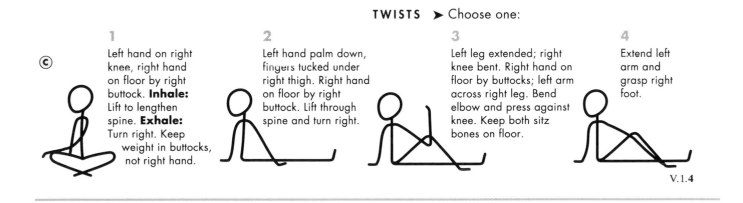

1 Left hand on right knee, right hand on floor by right buttock. **Inhale:** Lift to lengthen spine. **Exhale:** Turn right. Keep weight in buttocks, not right hand.

2 Left hand palm down, fingers tucked under right thigh. Right hand on floor by right buttock. Lift through spine and turn right.

3 Left leg extended; right knee bent. Right hand on floor by buttocks; left arm across right leg. Bend elbow and press against knee. Keep both sitz bones on floor.

4 Extend left arm and grasp right foot.

V.1.**4**

YOGA MUDRA VARIATION

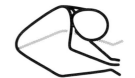

Sit with outer borders of feet on floor, hip-width apart, knees bend out. Hands or forearms on floor between legs. Let head hang. • OPTION: If sitting cross-legged is uncomfortable, use this position for other seated postures.

V.1.**5**

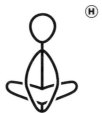

BADDHA KONASANA: COBBLER'S POSE

Place soles of feet together. Interlace fingers and hold under toes. Roll shoulders down from ears, inside of elbows toward ceiling. Lower knees toward floor.

V.2.**1**

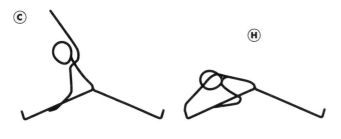

LEGS-WIDE-APART

Right thumb under right knee, palm up. **Inhale:** Lift left arm to ceiling. **Exhale:** Lower left hand to right toes. **Inhale:** Sweep left arm up, right arm raises. **Exhale:** Lower both arms.

V.2.**2**

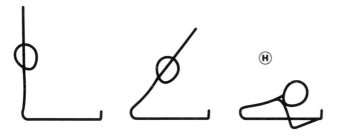

PASCHIMOTTANASANA: PASCIMATANASANA

Inhale: Raise arms. **Exhale:** Fold over legs. (Let knees give to release them and then restraighten.) Erratic breath signifies overwork. Relinquish your extension until breath is normal, then sink with each exhalation.

V.2.**3**

PARIPURNA NAVASANA: BOAT

Sitting on buttocks, lift legs until toes are above head. Fxtend arms at shoulder level, palms facing, outside legs. Keep spine lifting through top of head.

➤ Build to one minute each.

ARDHA NAVASANA: HALF BOAT

Interlace fingers, place hands behind head, point elbows toward feet, tuck chin to throat. Roll slightly behind sitz bones, lift legs until toes are in alignment with crown of head. (This position is much lower than boat and will be experienced in the abdomen; boat will be felt more in thighs.)

V.2.**4**

Ⓒ

If head is not on floor, keep arms in front of body, palms on floor near one another; bend elbows as possible out to side. Let head hang.

If forehead is on floor, hold right wrist with left hand behind back.

YOGA MUDRA

Sit cross-legged. Fold forward.

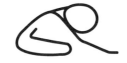 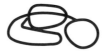

V.2.**5**

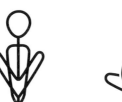

BUTTERFLY

Soles of feet together. Interlace fingers and hold under toes. **Exhale:** Lift knees. **Inhale:** Lower knees. (The Monarchs float through Morro Bay in great profusion in the fall.)

V.3.**1**

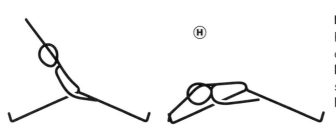

LEGS-WIDE-APART

Right palm faces upward under left leg. **Inhale:** Lift left arm to ceiling. **Exhale:** Grasp right toes with left hand. **Inhale:** Lift left arm toward ceiling and then lower to shoulder level as right arm raises to shoulder level. **Exhale:** Lower both arms.

V.3.**2**

PASCHIMOTTANASANA VARIATION

Place hands over toes, chest on thighs. Extend legs as far as possible keeping thighs and chest in contact.

V.3.**3**

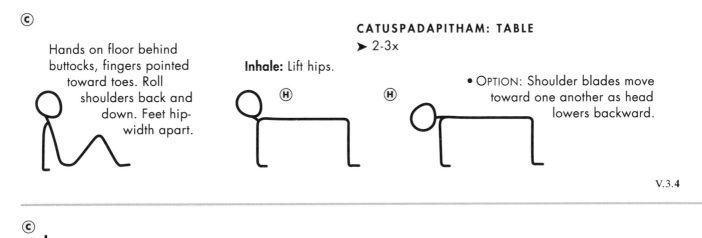

CATUSPADAPITHAM: TABLE
➤ 2-3x

Hands on floor behind buttocks, fingers pointed toward toes. Roll shoulders back and down. Feet hip-width apart.

Inhale: Lift hips.

• OPTION: Shoulder blades move toward one another as head lowers backward.

V.3.**4**

PASCHIMOTTANASANA: SEATED FORWARD BEND

Lift arms overhead alongside ears. **Inhale:** Extend. **Exhale:** Lower body and arms slightly to next stretch. Continue process 4-6 breaths then lower arms, hold position and breathe. **Inhale:** Lift arms and body. **Exhale:** Release.

V.3.**5**

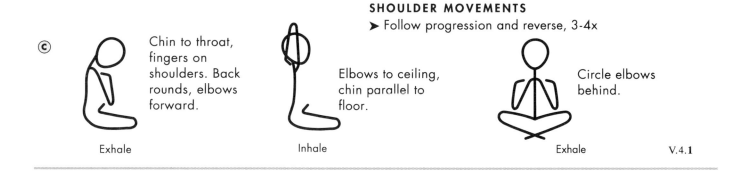

SHOULDER MOVEMENTS
➤ Follow progression and reverse, 3-4x

© Chin to throat, fingers on shoulders. Back rounds, elbows forward.

Exhale

Elbows to ceiling, chin parallel to floor.

Inhale

Circle elbows behind.

Exhale

V.4.**1**

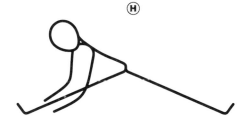

Ⓗ

PARIVRTTA JANU SIRSASANA
Right leg extended, left knee bent. Right little finger up, grasping ball of right foot; left little finger at right little toe (hand grasping outer border of foot). Rotate body and head as far as possible toward ceiling.

V.4.**2**

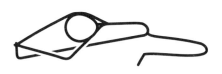

Ⓗ

LEGS-WIDE-APART
Hands on either side of leg. Fold forward; lower belly to thigh, then chest, then head. (Only lower head if chest is down.) Look down. Extend spine through top of head toward instep.

V.4.**3**

Ⓗ

UPAVISTA KONASANA: LEGS-WIDE-APART
Forward bend. Let belly lead chest to floor. Keep feet flexed, legs extend out of hip sockets.

V.4.**4**

UBHAYA PADANGUSTHASANA

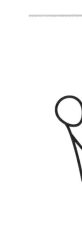

Balance on buttocks. Place hands under knees. Extend and rebend each leg. Extend both legs. Continue elongating spine.

Ⓗ

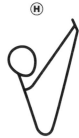

• OPTION: Interlace fingers and loop hands over soles of feet and straighten knees.

Then bring head to knees.

V.4.**5**

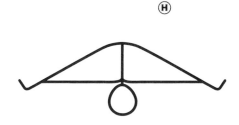

Ⓒ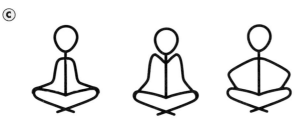

MOCKINGBIRD
Rest hands on knees. **Exhale:** Shrug shoulders. Inhale: Lower shoulders and lead with elbows down and to side.
➤ 4-6x

V.5.**1**

Ⓒ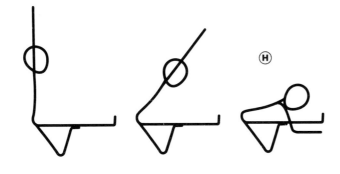

MAHAMUDRA
Extend left leg; bend right knee and place foot against left thigh; left hand near buttocks, fingers toward feet; chin to throat. Hold left leg (or toes) with right hand, keep right shoulder down. **Inhale:** Extend through spine. **Exhale:** Maintain extension. ➤ 3-6 breaths • OPTION: Place right hand on left foot, left hand on top of right. Keep shoulders down.

V.5.**2**

JANU SIRSASANA
Extend left leg; bend right knee and place foot against left thigh. **Inhale:** Raise arms. **Exhale:** Fold over left leg. Feel crown of head extending toward instep.

V.5.**3**

Ⓒ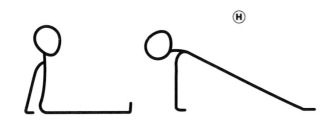

PURVATANASANA: INCLINED PLANE
Extend legs. Place hands on floor behind buttocks, fingers pointing toward toes. **Inhale:** Lift buttocks off floor. Keep feet flat. Face continues toward feet or turns to ceiling as shoulders roll down further. ➤ 2-3x

V.5.**4**

Ⓒ

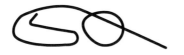

YOGA MUDRA VARIATION
Fold forward. Walk fingers away from body, elbows off floor.

V.5.**5**

SAVASANA CORPSE POSE
FINAL RELAXATION

■ While you are in Savasana your neuromuscular system can integrate the input it received during the active part of your practice. Savasana is the true finale of any practice session.

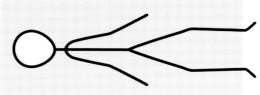

■ Lie on your back.
A folded blanket or a pillow under your knees will ease your back. Put a folded blanket or pillow under your head, if you wish.

■ Separate your legs about 18". Let your ankles and hips roll open.

■ Arms 8-10" from the sides of your body, palms facing the ceiling. Roll shoulders down and away from ears.
OPTION: Sit on a chair. Feet flat on the floor, back straight. Rest hands on thighs.

■ Allow your eyes to close.

■ Feel your body becoming heavier and heavier. Begin by directing your mind down into your toes. Then focus on each area of your body to the top of your head. Suggest to each part that it open, relax and release. As you relax more fully, your pulse, respiration and brain waves will all slow. Feel your body becoming warm and soft. After you have completed the relaxation of your body, watch your breath move in and out of your nostrils.
OPTION: Be the "observer" and watch, without attachment, the flow of thoughts through your mind.

■ For some, this is the most difficult asana of all. Encourage yourself with quiet, positive thoughts about ease, warmth, and openness to remain in savasana for 5-15 minutes. Often you will experience a deep feeling of peacefulness which will last for many hours after your practice has ended.

SPECIAL MOVEMENTS

For Your Hands

- Sit comfortably.
- Keep your shoulders relaxed.
- Do all or some of the following movements.
- Be sure to **continue breathing** throughout the exercises.

1. Palms face ceiling. Fold one finger at a time to palms, beginning with thumb. When all are folded, reopen hands. ➤ 3-4x

2. Palms face ceiling. Roll fingers toward palms beginning with little fingers. When all fingers are rolled in, rotate wrists so palms face floor and then return to beginning position. ➤ 6x

3. Palms face one another, fingers point to ceiling. Rotate thumbs. ➤ 6x each direction

4. Make loose fists and rotate hands. ➤ 6x each direction

5. Fold thumb and forefinger to form an O. Then stretch both fingers open as wide as possible. Follow same procedure with middle, ring and little fingers and back again. ➤ 3x each hand

6. Gently press fingers backwards with the opposite hand.

7. Massage each hand from the heel of the hand to the finger tips with the opposite hand.

SPECIAL MOVEMENTS

For Your Ankles

1 Assume one of these positions and circle ankles in both directions.

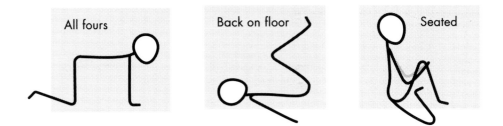

All fours

Back on floor

Seated

2 Sit with legs extended, about hip-width apart.
- Point toes, then flex feet. ➤ 6x
- Rotate ankles, turning toes out to side and then towards each other. ➤ 6x
- Turn toes toward each other, rotating thighs inward. In this position, point toes and then flex feet. ➤ 6x

3 Stand with feet about hip-width apart. Return to neutral position (feet flat on floor) between each of the following movements.
- Stand on heels, toes up.
- Stand on toes, heels up.
- Stand on outer borders of feet.
- Bend knees and stand on inner borders of feet.
  ➤ 4-6x

SPECIAL MOVEMENTS

For Your Feet

1 Stand on one foot with knee bent and roll a tennis ball underneath the other foot, applying as much pressure as you wish. After awhile, stand on both feet and feel the effects of the massage. • Repeat with the other foot.

2 Tuck toes and sit with buttocks on heels. • To release, come forward on hands and knees, extend toes on floor; then gently beat tops of feet against the floor.

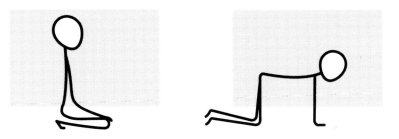

3 Massage the soles of your feet with your hands, working deeply with your thumbs. Consult a book on reflexology for further information.

4 Interlace fingers of right hand with toes of left foot (palm faces sole of foot). Use right thumb to massage. Also use fingers to massage the top of your foot.

5 As the pièce de résistance: with soles facing each other, interlace your toes.

SPECIAL MOVEMENTS

For Your Neck and Shoulders

■ Sit comfortably.
■ All of these movements should be done very slowly.

1 Turn your head from side to side, keeping chin parallel to the floor.
➤ 4 rounds each movement
- Lead with your chin.
- Lead with your ear.
- Lead with the energy body just outside of your face.

2 Nod "yes." Raise chin slightly higher than shoulder level and then fold it to your throat. ➤ 6x

3 Rest hands on knees. Circle shoulders in both directions.
➤ 6x each direction

4 • Turn head once to the right and once to the left, keeping chin parallel to the floor.

- Firmly grasp back of neck with right hand (hold muscles on both sides of neck). Imagine a spot in front of your nose and with your nose circle it (tiny circles). Circle for 3 breaths. Stop circling, slowly release grip and gently pull hand across neck and over right shoulder.

- Then, grasp neck with left hand and repeat, circling in the opposite direction. When you have completed 3 breaths, release grip and gently pull hand across neck and over left shoulder. Turn head carefully to the right and then to the left, keeping chin parallel to the floor. Notice the increase in your mobility.

SPECIAL MOVEMENTS

For Your Face

1   Open your mouth as wide as you can.

2   Smile a hard smile, pulling your lips toward your ears.

3   Make a very long 0, letting your upper lip fold over your upper teeth.

4   Purse your lips. Move them to the right and then to the left 2 times and then back to the center.

5   Form a long 0.

6   Open wide.

7   Smile.

Do not do eye movements with contact lens in your eyes.

1   Squeeze your eyes tightly and release, 2-3 times.

2   Flicker your eyelids open and shut rapidly. Let your eyes come to a gentle close.

3   Lift your eyebrows toward your hairline and release.

4   Squeeze your eyebrows toward the bridge of your nose and release.

5   Reach your eyebrows toward your ears and release.

6   Make faces using as many muscles as you can and then release.

■   These movements are a wonderful addition to Savasana (p. 77). Use them to relax the muscles of your face, either at the beginning of Savasana or after you have traveled through your body up to your head.

1

Stand.

Inhale

- This sequence of movements can: begin your practice, be practiced after Segment I, be your entire practice, or be omitted.
- To complete a round, follow these pictures in order. Then repeat the entire sequence, stepping back in #5 pose with the left foot and stepping forward with the left foot in #10 pose.
- Do 1-12 rounds.

2

Exhale

Namaste: palms together, fingers up in front of chest.

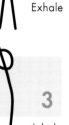

3

Inhale

Lift arms from side, leading up with backs of hands; rotate arms so palms face overhead. Then backward bend.

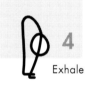

4

Exhale

Forward bend: hands beside feet, fingers aligned with toes. Bend knees if necessary.

5

Inhale

Large step back with right foot, lower knee to floor. Palms flat or fingers on floor.

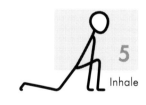

6

Hold breath

Board position: toes tucked, arms straight. Keep body and head in one line.

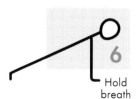

7

Exhale

Knees, chest and chin or forehead to floor.

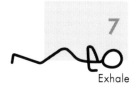

8

Inhale

Upward Facing Dog: toes tucked or rest on tops of feet, knees and thighs off floor. Roll shoulders back, press chest forward between arms.

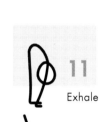

9

Exhale

Downward Facing Dog: palms on floor, fingers point straight ahead. Stretch the backs of your legs through your heels.

10

Inhale

Right foot forward between hands. Left knee on floor.

11

Exhale

Step in with left foot and hang or bring head to knees.

12

Inhale

Lift with flat back to standing. Bend knees if necessary.

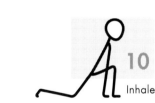

13

Exhale

Lower arms from side to Namaste.

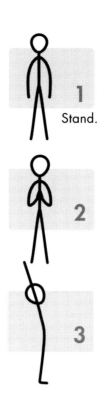

1 Stand.

MODIFIED SUN SALUTATION
- Breathing: Inhale; move into next position on exhalation.
- You can use this breathing technique for the traditional Sun Salutation, too.

2 Namaste: palms together, fingers up in front of chest.

3 Lift arms from side. Slight back bend.

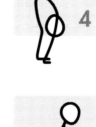

4 Forward bend: hands beside feet, fingers aligned with toes. Bend knees if necessary.

5 Large step back with right foot, lower knee to floor. Fingertips on floor.

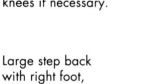

6 Board position: toes tucked, palms flat on floor, arms straight. Keep body and head in one line.

7 All fours.

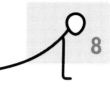

8 Upward Facing Dog: toes tucked under, knees and thighs off floor.

9 Downward Facing Dog: knees can bend.

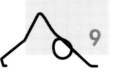

10 Bend knees and walk halfway toward hands so you can take weight on your feet and release your hands. Hang in forward bend.

11 Come up 2/3 of the way, bending elbows and knees to protect your back (keep weight in thighs).

12 Come to standing. Slight back bend.

13 Lower arms from side to Namaste.

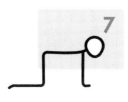

A PRACTICE SESSION AGAINST THE WALL

• This can be an entire practice. Breathe while holding poses.

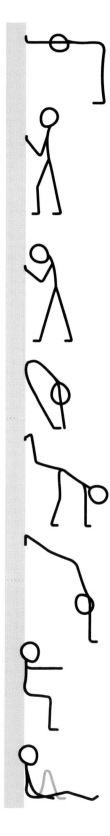

1
Hands on wall at hip height. Straighten arms and extend back.

2
One foot forward, several inches from wall. Bend elbows, place hands on wall. **Inhale:** Arch back, lift head, bend front leg.

Exhale: Round back, straighten leg, lower chin. (Spine leads, head follows.)
➤ 4-6x each side

3
Buttocks against wall, feet 8-10" away. Hang forward.

4
Back facing wall. Hands on floor shoulder-width apart. Spread fingers to form wide base. Place ball of foot as high on wall as you can.

Place other foot on wall. **Do not sway back.**

5
Half squat. Head, shoulders and buttocks against wall, feet flat on floor. ➤ 2-3x

6
Slide down wall. Release legs and rest.

7
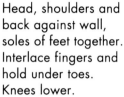
Downward Facing Dog. Thumbs and forefingers spread against wall. ➤ 2-3x

8
Head, shoulders and back against wall, soles of feet together. Interlace fingers and hold under toes. Knees lower.

9
Face wall, legs wide apart, feet against the wall. Legs stretch.

10
Same position as #9. Right hand on floor by buttock, left hand on right thigh. Twist right. Reverse hands, twist left.

11
Lie on back, bend knees, feet flat against wall. Rest.

12
Same position as #11. Bridge: lift buttocks, leave head, shoulders and arms on floor.
➤ 2-3x

13
Roll down and rest with head, back and arms on floor and legs extended up wall.

INDEX

INDEX

RECOMMENDED REFERENCES

▓ Couch, Jean. **The Runner's Yoga Book.** "A Balanced Approach to Fitness." Berkeley, California: Rodmell Press, 1990.

▓ Iyengar, B.K.S. **Light on Yoga.** New York: Schocken Books, Revised Edition 1977.

▓ Rawlinson, Ian. **Yoga for the West.** Sebastopol, California: CRCS Publications, 1987.

▓ Schonfeld, David. **Yoga for a Better Life.** Wheaton, Illinois: Theosophical Publishing House, 1980.

Connie Weiss is available for
workshops and can be reached through
Lurie Lane Publishing, P.O. Box 893,
Morro Bay, California 93442

▓

(805) 772-2347